NUTRITION
For Athletes

*P*hysical *F*itness
and
*S*ports *M*edicine

Below is a listing of the currently available (or soon to be available) books in this new series:

- *Strength-Training Principles* by Ellington Darden, Ph.D.
- *Olympic Athletes Ask Questions About Exercise and Nutrition* by Ellington Darden, Ph.D.
- *How to Lose Body Fat* by Ellington Darden, Ph.D.
- *Soccer Fitness* by David Ponsonby, M.Ed., and Ellington Darden, Ph.D.
- *7 Steps to Heart and Lung Fitness* by Richard Rylander Blide, M.D.
- *How Your Muscles Work: Featuring Nautilus Training Equipment* by Ellington Darden, Ph.D.
- *Care and Conditioning of the Pitching Arm* (For Little League Baseball) by Fred L. Allman, Jr., M.D.
- *The Week-End Athlete's Guide to Sports Medicine: Lower Body* by James D. Key, M.D.
- *Nutrition For Athletes* by Ellington Darden, Ph.D.
- *Conditioning For Football* by Ellington Darden, Ph.D.
- *The Week-End Athlete's Guide to Sports Medicine: Upper Body* by James D. Key, M.D.

Write to Anna Publishing for a complete description of titles, publication dates, and prices.

NUTRITION
For Athletes

Ellington Darden, Ph.D.

Director of Research
Nautilus Sports/Medical Industries
Executive Program Director
Athletic Center of Atlanta, Georgia

Anna Publishing, Inc.
Winter Park, Florida 32792

Cover Art by
Inverse Reflections (Scott LeGear)

Copyright © 1978 by

Anna Publishing, Inc.
Winter Park, Florida

2nd Printing

Library of Congress Catalog Card Number: 77-076070

International Standard Book Number: 0-89305-014-8

Printed in U.S.A.

Contents

Introduction

For ten years, from 1959 to 1969, I was a firm believer in high-protein supplements and vitamin pills as well as other so-called "health foods." I took vitamin B_{12} for endurance, wheat germ oil for energy, garlic for purifying the blood, kelp tablets for muscle definition, and vitamin B_6 for strength. At the same time I avoided white bread, carbonated drinks, ice cream, and most carbohydrate foods.

Why did I follow this diet? Mainly because I was convinced that the quickest way to become a superior athlete was to follow such a program of eating. Where did I get these beliefs? The majority of them came from the popular physical fitness and health magazines. According to the periodicals, most of the recent champions had followed such a program. It was not unusual to read a testimony that a certain diet was at least 75 percent responsible for their being a winner.

I never questioned these concepts until I entered graduate school at Florida State University. In fact, most of the time I was trying to find new ways or more concentrated protein supplements to be certain that I was consuming over 300 grams of protein a day.

During my first year at FSU, I attended a graduate seminar at which Dr. Harold E. Schendel gave a two-hour lecture on the role of nutrition in physical fitness. Dr. Schendel was professor of nutrition at FSU, but had spent four years previously in Africa and elsewhere directing research on problems of protein malnutrition. He has published over 70 papers in this and related areas.

After our initial meeting, we spent many hours discussing what effect various foods and eating habits have on athletic performance. To say the least, Dr. Schendel disagreed with most of my nutritional concepts and did not believe that my special eating habits or diet were necessary, beneficial, or even safe. His point was that an athlete did **not** require large amounts of vitamins, proteins, or any "health foods." Since I was so convinced about the value of my diet, he didn't argue with me. Rather, he suggested that I read the research literature on this subject and decide for myself what was the best diet for an athlete.

Needless to say, I was not convinced by Dr. Schendel's ideas. After all, his knowledge was mostly theoretical, but I was actually eating a special diet and "knew" about its value. I was a hard training athlete who was constantly trying to increase strength and endurance and I was not about to change my training program because of any university professor or research work done with rats. The physical fitness magazines seemed to make sense to me when they promoted the sale of their food supplements. Therefore, dietary supplementation was more than justified; it was essential!

Rather than spend time arguing this point, Dr. Schendel suggested I conduct an experiment on myself. We decided to determine if an athlete in hard training could use the massive amounts of protein I was eating. We agreed that if my body could not use this amount of protein (but broke it down and discarded its end products in the urine), then it surely must not require it.

In order to do this, we kept precise records of my caloric intake (including supplements) and caloric expenditure (including all training) for a two-month period. We varied the protein intake from less than 100 grams a day to more than 380 grams, most of which was obtained from a 90 percent protein powder. All of my urine was collected during the entire period and analyzed for excreted protein end products.

The result of this two-month study started me thinking in a different direction. To my surprise, whenever I consumed over approximately 80 grams of protein a day, it was excreted. (My protein needs according to the Recommended Dietary Allowances, at a bodyweight of 215 pounds, were 77 grams a day.) Furthermore, my body weight remained relatively stationary throughout the entire period. No difference in strength was noted, regardless of the amount of protein consumed. In fact, when I went off the massive protein diet I noticed an additional surge of energy. This may have been due to the fact that several of my body's tissues and organs must work very hard to metabolize excessive amounts of protein and my body was freed from this cost or burden when I stopped eating the protein.

If my body was not utilizing these massive amounts of protein, was it possible that the same thing could be true when I consumed more than the Recommended Dietary Allowances of various vitamins and minerals? Additional research revealed this was exactly what was happening.

These facts from my own personal experience have convinced me that many protein, vitamin, and mineral supplements, and "health foods" on the market are not being sold or promoted to meet the nutritional requirements of athletes, but rather to make a few people very rich.

Now, approximately nine years after this eye-opening experience, I'm more convinced than ever that food supplements are not necessary for optimum performance. In fact, similar conclusions have been drawn by nutritional scientists since the 1930s and have been repeatedly confirmed over and over again. But it certainly does not follow that this same lesson has been learned by other athletes. On the contrary, most athletes are constantly on the lookout for a magic food, pill, potion, or dietary regimen that will change them overnight from a mediocre performer into a world champion.

In the light of my own experience, I can certainly understand why they make such mistakes ... after all, I continued making the exact same mistakes for over ten years.

So it was a hard lesson for me to learn . . . and perhaps I'm expecting a bit much of other athletes when I expect them to learn the same lesson quickly and easily. Some athletes do, but some don't . . . and some apparently never will, remaining firmly if falsely convinced that food supplements are necessary for optimum performance. Yet, the facts show that all that's needed for optimum athletic performance is a well-balanced diet composed of a variety of nutritious food from your corner grocery or neighborhood supermarket.

But, when a champion athlete comes on the scene with an outstanding degree of speed, strength, endurance, or ability and loudly proclaims himself an "expert," and points to his own performance as undeniable proof that certain food supplements are primarily responsible . . . then I suppose it's perfectly natural for many athletes to pay attention to his words.

Perfectly natural it may be, but it's almost always a mistake. I have yet to meet a single example of such an athlete who has even a basic understanding of the actual cause and effect relationship involved in nutrition and performance. Such people are simply statistical standouts, genetic freaks . . . and have produced their obvious results in spite of their nutritional beliefs, rather than as a result of any real knowledge.

This is not to say, however, that nutrition is not important in athletic performance. While most of the alleged benefits of special diets and supplements are not accurately stated, correct nutrition for the athlete can mean the difference between having enough stamina and tiring halfway through a game; or between a sense of well-being and a feeling of not being up to par. It can also make the difference between winning and losing. Of course, factors other than diet can affect performance, but taking nutrition for granted or the indiscriminate use of dietary supplements, may produce an unnecessary handicap or be dangerous to health.

Nutrition For Athletes is divided into three parts. Part 1 examines some common nutritional beliefs that many athletes adhere to ... which are, in fact myths. A bit of humor is added in the form of cartoons by Dr. George Moudry of the Sports Medicine Clinic, Atlanta, Georgia. For athletes who want to know more about nutrition, Part 2 summarizes the important nutrients in foods. In Part 3, you'll find special diets, exercise routines, and all the facts and figures necessary to gain solid bodyweight.

Part I

Myths
and
Truths

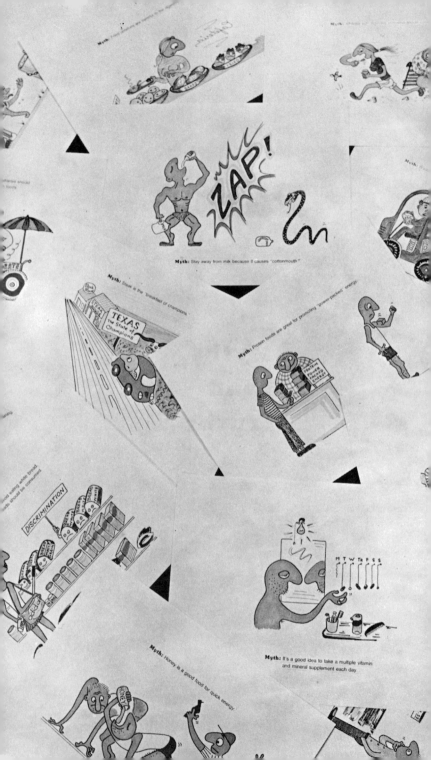

Myths and Truths

Myths are created from ignorance ... total or partial. The dictionary defines a myth as "a traditional story of unknown authorship ... serving to explain some phenomenon." It usually represents a falsified description, or at best, an incomplete one.

In the case of nutrition, it's easy to understand why ignorance has been perpetuated. Historically, nutrition is a youngster in the scientific community, having been recognized as a distinct discipline only in 1934. As a result, we find many self-proclaimed experts in nutrition, who are "experts" simply because they've eaten food all their lives! Now, combine this with the sports world, where it's common knowledge that coaches and athletes are some of the world's worst faddists, and it isn't surprising that we've got quite a list of food-related myths.

Truth, on the other hand, has been pursued by philosophers and scientists since days of ancient Greece. Turning to the dictionary, we find that truth is "the quality of being in accordance with experience, facts, or reality." The truth conforms with fact.

15

Tremendous progress in obtaining nutritional facts has been made within the past 50 years. The composition of most foods is now well known. The major changes that food components undergo in the body are fairly well understood. Although the total picture will probably never be clear, ample facts exist about how fats and carbohydrates are converted to energy, how protein is incorporated into body tissue, and how vitamins and minerals function. In addition, ample facts exist on why many nutritional practices and beliefs **don't** contribute to winning. All of these facts or truths have direct application to improving athletic performance.

In this book, evidence to combat myths will be presented from research undertaken not only in sports situations but from other areas as well. This information represents what we know at the present time, based on fact.

Myth: Most athletes should not be concerned about calories.

Truth: Calories do count, every one of them. Consume more calories than your body expends, and you'll gain fat; less calories, and you'll lose fat (there's approximately 3,500 calories in a pound of fat). This is in accordance with the law of conservation of energy which states that energy may be converted or transferred, but cannot be created or destroyed. In other words, the energy value of food eaten (minus the energy lost in the excreta) must equal the sum of the heat given off and the physical work done by the body. The unit measure of heat energy is the calorie, but surprisingly, few people actually know what a calorie really is.

A calorie (kilocalorie is actually the more appropriate term) is the amount of heat you would need to raise the temperature of one liter (a little more than a quart) of water one degree centigrade. To help you visualize that, 100 calories would raise the temperature of one liter of water from freezing level to boiling.

Myth: Steak is the "breakfast of champions."

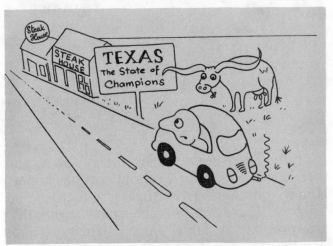

Truth: Thick, juicy steaks have been a training table staple for many years. This was especially prevalent when I was growing up in Texas during the 1950s and 1960s. Even today, many coaches and trainers believe that there's a corollary between red meat and strength and endurance.

Scientific research has repeatedly shown that steak, which contains protein and fat, is not as efficient in supplying energy for athletic performance as food rich in carbohydrates. The ideal diet for athletes should be composed of 59 percent carbohydrate, 28 percent fat, and 13 percent protein.

Myth: Honey is a good food for quick energy.

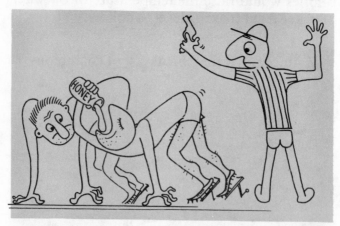

Truth: There are no quick-energy foods, and there's nothing magic about eating honey. Honey contains two sugars, glucose and fructose. These are the same simple sugars that are present in table sugar. Honey is not significantly superior to other common sweets, although it does contain a greater percentage of fructose. Unfortunately dietary quacks have falsely promoted honey as a sweet that is better tolerated than other sugars. This is not true.

Taken in large quantities, honey can produce several detrimental effects. Excess amounts of honey (or other similar sweets), tend to draw fluid from other parts of the body into the gastrointestinal tract. This shift in fluids may add to the problem of dehydration in long distance events, where sweat loss can affect performance. The body also may rebel if the sugar intake is too high. A concentrated sugar solution may cause extra distention in the stomach, and the evacuation mechanism may be impaired. Problems such as cramps, nausea, and diarrhea can occur. Therefore, no more than 50 grams of sugar (3 rounded tablespoons) in a liquid should be taken in any one-hour period. Even then, these foods do not seem to improve performance in short-term events.

Myth: Pre-competition meals for athletes should consist of carbohydrate-rich foods.

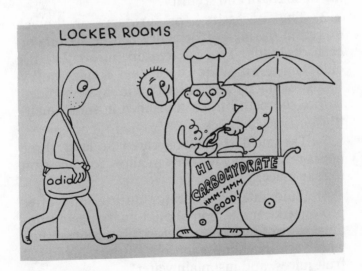

Truth: What you eat on the day of competition has very little to do with the production of energy for that day. (The exception to this rule is athletes that compete in non-stop, marathon-type events. They can benefit from pre-event meals composed of carbohydrate-rich foods, as well as several days of carbohydrate loading). Nutritional scientists have found that it ordinarily takes from two to fourteen days for the food you eat to actually be utilized in the form of energy. Nevertheless, the following guidelines should be considered in planning pre-competition meals:

1. Energy intakes should be adequate to ward off any feelings of hunger or weakness during competition. Although the food eaten prior to competition has little to do with immediate energy expenditure, it can give the athlete a feeling of strength and security.

2. The necessity for urinary or bowel excretion during performance can be serious or even disabling. For this reason, meals that include large amounts of protein foods, bulky foods, or highly spiced foods should be avoided before competition, or consumed in small quantities.

3. The meal should be eaten at least three hours prior to starting time to allow for digestion to take place.

4. Fluid intakes prior to, during, and after prolonged competition should guarantee an optimal state of hydration. This can be accomplished with various saline solutions, "thirst drinks," fruit juices, and just plain water!

5. And finally, the pre-competition meal should include food that the athlete is familiar with . . . food that will "make him win." Remember, eating can be as much psychological as it is physiological.

Myth: You should refrain from eating sweets while in training.

Truth: Sugars and starches furnish the most efficient fuel for muscular work. In fact, from 50 to 60 percent of a athlete's diet should be composed of carbohydrate-rich foods: fruits, vegetables, breads, cereals, and sweets. There is no good reason why athletes in training should not eat moderate amounts of sweets or sugars. Of course an athlete in training needs the other elements of a balanced diet also.

Myth: Fried potatoes are harmful to the digestive tract.

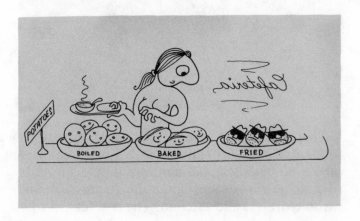

Truth: All greasy foods are digested slowly because fat retards the emptying time of the stomach, but this does no harm to a normal digestive tract. Most fats are digested at about the same rate whether they are in the form of butter, margarine, salad dressing, shortening, or cooking oils used to fry foods, such as potatoes. As for potatoes, they are one of the most nutritious of all vegetables. Fried potatoes, therefore, are certainly not taboo for athletes.

Myth: Bread is a fattening food, so athletes should avoid it.

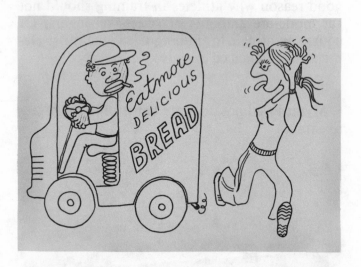

Truth: Bread is one of the most nutritious foods that athletes can eat. It is low in calories (about 60 per slice) and contains ample amounts of niacin, riboflavin, thiamine, iron, protein, carbohydrates, and calcium. The real reason why the majority of people relate bread to fattening food is not the bread itself, but what they put on it!

Myth: All athletes should avoid eating white bread. Only whole-grain breads should be consumed.

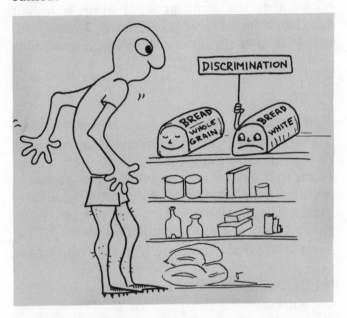

Truth: Basically, there are no significant differences between the nutritional quality of whole-grain bread and enriched white bread ... especially when you consider the cost of a loaf of each. Enriched white bread, when thiamine, niacin, riboflavin, and iron have been added, and when milk solids are used in baking, provides practically the same values of thiamine, niacin, and iron as whole-wheat bread. It also gives twice as much riboflavin, and a great deal more calcium because of the milk which is absent from whole-wheat bread. It's true that minute amounts of some nutrients like sodium, magnesium, and other trace elements are lost in milling white flour, but there are numerous other food sources of the lost nutrients. Therefore where bread is concerned, you can eat what appeals to you whether it be white, dark, French, Italian, etc., just as long as the label states "whole-grain," or "enriched."

Myth: Eating grapefruit helps you to burn fat.

Truth: There is nothing unique about grapefruit in regard to burning fat. In fact, there are **no foods** that oxidize or dissolve fat. Fat cannot be excreted from your body. As a result, something must be done with the extra energy sources you eat and there are only two possibilities:

(1) Your body can store it in the form of fat, or,

(2) It can oxidize it if demanded by cell or body need.

While grapefruit does not have any magical qualities, it's an excellent food to include in your diet. It's a good source of vitamin C, vitamin A, calcium, and several B vitamins.

Myth: In order to lose fat, you should drastically reduce your carbohydrate intake.

Truth: Fad diets (and that's exactly what low-carbohydrate diets are) may cause a loss of weight, but generally speaking, most of the weight does not come from fat cells. Reducing your carbohydrate consumption to under 60 grams a day can cause a loss of water, which usually comes from your muscles rather than fat (there's very little water in fat). Instead of drastically reducing your carbohydrate intake, you should moderately cut back on **all foods.** There are no quick and easy ways **to lose fat!** Losing fat is hard . . . very hard. Nutritionists recommend that you set a realistic goal in losing fat of from one to two percent of your bodyweight per week. In this fashion you can be sure that the weight you lose is fat.

Myth: Bee pollen tablets offer a tremendous breakthrough in helping an athlete run faster and farther.

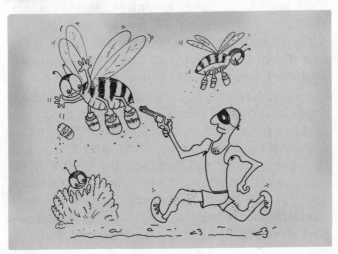

Truth: The athletic world can thank the Finns for publicizing bee pollen. It all started in 1972 when Finland's Lasse Viren won the 5,000- and 10,000-meter runs in Munich and began buzzing the news about pollen tablets.

When Viren repeated his successes in Montreal in 1976, health-food companies decided to make it available ... at a cost of as much as $45 per pound. The cost is a result of not only it's "magical" properties, but the way it is gathered. The pollen is gathered by placing wire brushes around the entrances to the bee hives. As the bees obtain nectar from flowers, pollen collects on their bodies. And when the bees return to their hives, the wire brushes act as a foot scraper, sort of like you'd use on a muddy day before going into your front door.

This very fine powder is then collected and manufactured into tablets or pellets. Bee pollen in tablet form contains, according to the U.S. distributor, all the essential amino acids, vitamins A and most of the B complex, and many trace minerals. There are no magic nutrients in bee pollen that can't be obtained in conventional, less expensive foods.

Recent research at Louisiana State University conducted by Dr. John C. Wells' group, showed that bee pollen has no effect on the performance of runners and swimmers. When confronted with this evidence, the American distributor noted that the LSU study used bee pollen from France, and not the full-potency pollen from England, which naturally he sold! The distributor also said that if you consumed a well-balanced diet, bee

26

pollen would not be beneficial. This is just another of the many myths that surround the athletic world.

Myth: Taking lecithin regularly is a good preventive measure against heart disease.

Truth: Lecithin is the natural emulsifier found in egg yolks and soybeans and is sold in capsule and powder form at "health food" stores. It has long been publicized in health magazines as an antidote to too high blood cholesterol and heart disease. Evidence shows that lecithin cannot dissolve the plaques in the blood vessels that contribute to heart attacks. Unfortunately, solving the problems associated with high blood cholesterol concentrations and heart disease are much more complex than a simple feeding of lecithin.

Myth: Stay away from hamburgers during training.

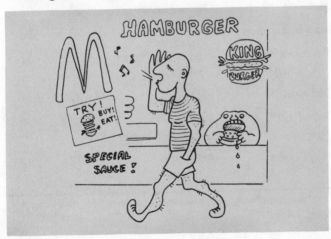

Truth: A hamburger with all the trimmings (lettuce, tomatoes, onions, cheese, salad dressing, as well as lean meat and bread), is a fairly well-balanced meal. There's no good reason why athletes could not consume hamburgers several times a week. The same thing could be said about other foods purchased at fast-food chains.

As examples, let's examine the number of calories and grams of protein present in typical selections from well known fast-food restaurants.

Fast Food Nutrition Chart

Fast-Food Restaurants	Menu Items	Protein (in grams)	Calories
A&W	Super Papa Burger	19	448
Burger Chef	Super Chef	23	423
Burger King	Whopper	29	563
Dairy Queen	Super Brazier	43	732
Hardee's	Deluxe Huskee	32	635
Jack-In-The-Box	Jumbo Jack	28	558
Kentucky Fried Chicken	2-piece Box Munch with roll	32	451
McDonald's	Big Mac	27	543
Pizza Hut	½ Small Pizza Supreme (thin crust)	42	799
Roy Rogers	Roast Beef Sandwich	22	292

All data compiled by Jacobs-Winston Laboratories Inc., New York, N.Y.

If you eat at a fast-food chain regularly, it would be wise to make sure that your other meals include such nutritious foods as beans, dairy products, and a wide variety of fruits and vegetables.

Myth: Table sugar should be avoided like the plague.
Truth: Sugar does not contain a single harmful substance. Nothing is added in refining that is toxic to the body.

The problem with refined sugar is that it is dehydrated cane and beet juice, which dehydration results in concentrated calories. And sugar's calories contain no other nutrients like vitamins or minerals.

Nutritionists would prefer that you get most of your carbohydrates from foods that also supply vitamins, minerals, and bulk. Fruits, vegetables, and breads, for example, are rich in carbohydrates as well as many other useful nutrients.

Table sugar, therefore, should not be avoided "like the plague" ... but merely used in moderation.

Myth: Teenage athletes should drink at least two glasses of milk a day.
Truth: All athletes, not only teenagers, should consume several servings of dairy products each day, but not necessarily milk. Recent surveys

show that at least 30 million Americans suffer from milk intolerance, or more specifically, intolerance of a certain sugar in milk.

Milk contains lactose, a sugar which, as long as it stays in that form, is indigestible. But the small intestine produces an enzyme, lactase, which splits the lactose into simple sugars that are easily digested.

Intolerance develops when the body loses the capacity to produce adequate amounts of the enzyme. The undigested lactose then passes through the gut and causes disturbances, like abdominal bloating, cramps, and diarrhea.

If you have symptoms that might be related to milk intolerance, how can you tell for sure?

One way is for a physician to do a lactose-tolerance test. You consume a specified amount of milk and measurements are then made on a sample of blood. If you have plenty of the enzyme, the blood will temporarily contain high levels of sugar because the lactase is adequate to break down the milk sugar so it can be absorbed and get into the blood. Conversely, low blood levels point to intolerance.

You can also limit your milk intake or stop it entirely for about a week and see if your symptoms disappear.

People who have the problem can usually eat milk alternatives. Yogurt, hard cheeses, and similar dairy products have a lower lactose content because some of the sugar has fermented and changed during processing.

Or, there's a new product available, Lact-Aid, that can be added to a quart of milk. It is made from yeast and provides the missing or deficient lactase enzyme. Lact-Aid is available in packets at your local supermarket.

Myth: Drinking water during practice will upset an athlete's stomach; besides drinking water has a tendency to slow you down.

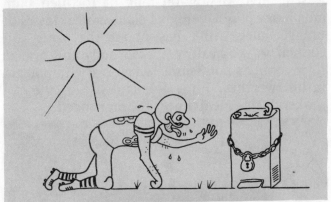

Truth: Prohibiting drinking water on the practice field has no physiological basis. Withholding liquids during hot, humid weather, in fact, makes an athlete very susceptible to one of the major heat syndromes: heat cramps, heat exhaustion, or the more serious and sometimes fatal heat stroke. Furthermore, dehydration causes fatigue, which in itself makes an athlete more vulnerable to injury.

All coaches, athletes, and even non-athletes should be informed of the necessity of drinking fluids before, during, and after all vigorous activity.

31

Myth: During hot weather, athletes should consume several salt tablets each day.

Truth: Taking salt tablets usually does more harm than good. Granted athletes need more salt during hot weather, but salt tablets have a tendency to irritate the stomach or be passed through the system completely undissolved. Dr. Lawrence E. Lamb recommends that in addition to drinking plenty of water, athletes should drink at least a quart of low-fat milk or fortified skim milk a day plus a couple of eight-ounce glasses of orange juice. Milk has about the same salt content as the healthy human body and orange juice contains potassium, which is also important in hot weather. Plus, a liberal use of the salt shaker during meal time is recommended.

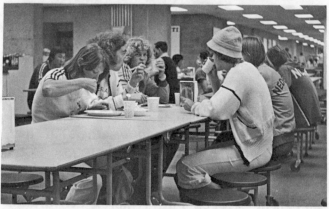

While in training, athletes should drink liberal amounts of water and other liquids.

Myth: All protein is alike.

Truth: Since body protein is composed of amino acid building blocks, you might think that all food is alike in terms of protein. But this is not true. Foods differ greatly in their content of amino acids.

The amino acids that must be provided by your foods are called "essential amino acids." These cannot be synthesized by your body, hence they must be provided by the food you eat. The other amino acids can be made by your body tissues.

In general, animal-source foods (beef, pork, eggs, milk, fish) provide adequate amounts of all the essential amino acids. Thus, relatively small quantities of animal-source protein each day should take care of your needs.

Myth: Large amounts of protein foods and protein supplements are especially important during intense training.

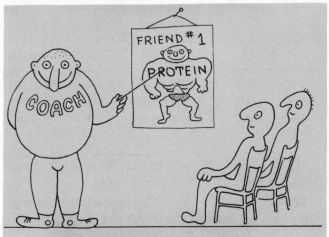

Truth: Contrary to what many Americans believe and contrary to what physical fitness and health magazines would have you believe, most Americans get more than enough protein. In fact you'd have to look long and hard to find **any** American athletes who are deficient in protein. Surveys show that numerous athletes consume four or five times their actual requirements. There are absolutely **no** health or performance benefits from excessive "high-protein" eating.

How much protein do you need? The following table was developed from the Recommended Dietary Allowances.

How Much Protein You Need

	Average Weight	For Protein Needs Multiply Weight by:	Average Protein Need
Child, 1-3	28 pounds	0.80	22 grams
Child, 4-6	44 pounds	0.70	31 grams
Child, 7-10	66 pounds	0.55	36 grams
Male, 11-14	97 pounds	0.45	44 grams
Male, 15-18	134 pounds	0.40	54 grams
Male, over 19	162 pounds	0.36	58 grams
Female, 11-14	97 pounds	0.45	44 grams
Female, 15-18	119 pounds	0.40	48 grams
Female, over 19	135 pounds	0.36	49 grams

Myth: Most of an athlete's protein foods should be eaten at the evening meal.

Truth: There's been a growing national tendency to crowd most of the day's protein foods into the evening meal. What's wrong with the above habit? The basic problem is that the cells must have all the amino acids continually available for building and repair.

The desirability of spreading protein intake during the day, so as to keep an adequate supply of essential amino acids always available is one of the reasons breakfast is considered such an important meal. But studies suggest that 50 percent of American children, and many athletes of all ages, eat breakfasts that are rated poor in protein. Skipping breakfast can eventually have a detrimental effect on athletic performance.

So practice eating a hearty, nutritious breakfast that contains some protein-rich foods.

Myth: Protein foods are great for promoting "power-packed" energy.

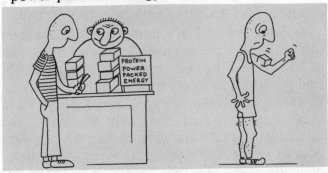

Truth: Although proteins can be used as energy sources if necessary, energy is almost always provided by carbohydrates and fats. These two nutrients are much preferred as energy sources, being more easily utilized in the body and less expensive than protein foods. The promotion of "power-packed" protein, therefore, is nothing more than a sales gimmick.

Myth: High-protein diets are a must for fat reduction.

Truth: First of all, proteins and carbohydrates have the same caloric value -- four calories per gram. Fats, on the other hand, provide nine calories per gram. A "high-protein" diet tends to be high in fat. People who go all out on high-protein reducing diets can easily wind up on a food plan in which 70 percent or more of the calories come from fat.

Then why are there so many testimonials for the benefit of protein diets? Because, they seem to work! One reason for this is that part of the weight loss on a high-protein diet is attributed to the fact that it causes minor nausea and loss of appetite. This leads to a reduced caloric intake.

Another reason is the human body encounters difficulty when it must use a great deal of protein as fuel. When the body breaks protein down for fuel purposes, there are waste products that must be removed by the kidneys. The kidneys flush these wastes out of the body as urine. The resulting unusual water loss, perhaps five to eight pounds in the first week, makes the dieter think he is losing fat. There is very little water in fat! Thus, the water comes from the muscles, vital organs, and extra-cellular fluid.

This is exactly what's happening with the wide variety of liquid protein supplements, amino acid supplements, and high-protein powders that are currently sweeping the country as the so-called "protein-sparing fast." The sad part, however, is that none of them cause long-term fat loss ... and many of the are actually dangerous.

Myth: Consuming large amounts of protein can't hurt your body.

Truth: Scientists have recently found that excessive amounts of dietary protein may be dangerous to your body. The metabolism and excretion on nonstorable protein loads impose serious stress and cause hypertrophy of several important organs, especially the liver and kidneys.

The current controversy over the liquid protein (amino acid) supplements, has frightened many people ... and rightly so. As of January 1978, government investigators suspect that at least 40 reported deaths may be linked to the diet that combines fasting with the use of the liquid. Most of the liquid protein diets sold over the counter aren't properly fortified with minerals, particularly potassium, a deficiency of which can lead to sudden death. The diet may also produce big shifts in body water and electrolytes, causing cardiac arrest. The diet was popularized by Robert Linn in his book, **The Last Chance Diet,** which was published in July 1976.

Prior to this date, however, athletes (especially bodybuilders and weightlifters) had been consuming the liquid protein supplements for years, hoping it would make them bigger and stronger. Fortunately, they were also consuming other foods. Scientists who have analyzed the dark syrupy liquids say they contain low quality, partly digested protein derived from cattle hides and tendons. Artificial flavor and saccharin are added to disguise the otherwise horrid taste.

Once again, there is no scientific evidence available that supports the popular idea that athletes require massive amounts of protein-rich foods, protein supplements (pills or powder), or liquid amino acids, as a result of strenuous activities.

Myth: Raw eggs should be added to a milk shake for additional nutrition.

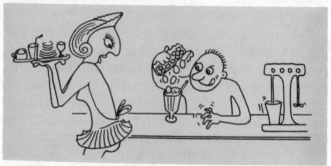

Truth: Although the addition of raw eggs can improve the flavor and nutritional value of a milk shake, this should be avoided because of the possibility of illness from contaminated eggs. Residual salmonella organism, which causes food poisoning, can remain on the outside of eggs even after washing. Invisible cracks in the shell may permit passage of the disease organism. Nutritionally, raw eggs are less desirable because they contain avidin (neutralized in cooking), which destroys biotin, a B vitamin. The usual methods of cooking eggs assure a safe product. Or, try adding eggs that are slightly soft boiled to your milk shake.

Myth: It's a good idea to take a multiple vitamin and mineral supplement each day.

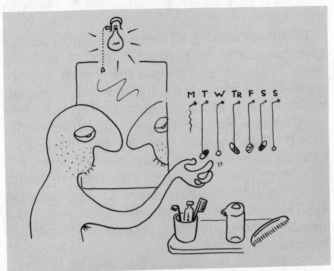

Truth: A recent commercial on TV shows an athletic-looking person explaining how he stays healthy. He says he watches his diet, gets plenty of exercise, and . . . "just to be sure" . . . takes a vitamin-mineral supplement each day.

This is the way we've come to expect the marketing of dietary supplements. They are promoted as an "insurance" policy to guarantee good health. The implication of such advertising has contributed to the myth that a balanced diet cannot provide adequate nutrients.

This is untrue. More is known about the nutrient content of food today than ever before. A balanced diet that meets the U.S. RDA requirements for vitamins A, B_1, B_2, C, and D will always provide the needed amounts of other vitamins, despite the claims of some people that these other vitamins are hard to find and therefore must be eaten in special foods or taken by pill.

In other words, all necessary nutrients are easily available in a sensible diet of ordinary foods. The sole exception is the case of iron for women. Approximately five percent of female athletes have excessive menstrual flows. Iron supplements may be necessary for those in this group. Although the consumption of a daily vitamin and mineral pill may cause no harm, it is possible that excessive amounts of some nutrients (like vitamins A and D) can be toxic. It's always a good idea to check with your personal physician before taking any vitamin and mineral supplement.

Myth: When taking vitamin supplements, be sure they're from natural rather than synthetic sources.

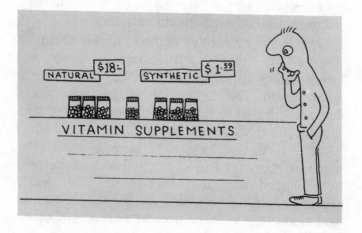

Truth: Basically there is no difference between natural and synthetic vitamins, except for the higher costs of the natural ones. Both have the same atoms in their molecules and are arranged in exactly the same way, which means their chemical behaviors are identical. A vitamin is a vitamin, period. The idea of selling natural vitamins as somehow better is a cleverly designed hoax.

Myth: Athletes should try their best to buy and consume organically grown fruits and vegetables.

Truth: Many athletes mistakenly believe that all organic foods are produced without pesticides and artificial fertilizers and that they are free of perservatives, hormones, and antibiotics. Unfortunately, there are no legal standards concerning organically grown foods. And there isn't even a consistent definition! "Organic" is not a synonym for "pure." In fact, the organic fertilizer of animal or human origin is the most likely to contain gastrointestinal parasites. Salmonella, which upsets more stomachs than probably anything else, is a frequent inhabitant of the gastrointestinal tract of animals and men. It represents a serious threat to the whole concept of "organically grown" ... especially if the foods are not washed or cooked prior to consumption. You should remember that the major danger in eating is still bacterial or parasitic contamination.

Myth: Fresh fruits and vegetables are nutritionally superior to frozen or canned fruits and vegetables.

Truth: Generally speaking, if "fresh" means locally grown, picked when ripe, and rushed to the market, then this statement is not a myth. But if "fresh" means harvested in California and shipped by truck to the East Coast ... or mid-December peaches from Chile, then canned or frozen produce is probably a better choice. Canned, frozen, and fresh ... each in its own way and its own season, has its drawbacks and its values. The best way to ensure proper nutrition is to eat a wide variety of all styles of fruits and vegetables.

Myth: Large doses of wheat germ oil will improve your stamina.

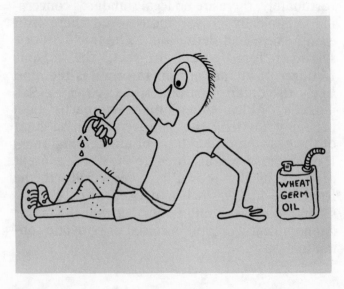

Truth: Wheat germ oil is rich in vitamin E, a necessary nutrient, but taking large amounts of it will not improve your stamina. Vitamin E is a fat-soluble nutrient which is important in certain glandular functions. It also acts as an anti-oxidant, thereby directly or indirectly participating in various oxidation-reduction reactions in the body. Because of these reactions, athletes have apparently assumed that taking large doses of wheat germ oil (or vitamin E) will improve their stamina. While taking large doses of wheat germ oil may not be harmful to the body, it is very expensive (over $5.00 a pint), is high in calories, and is not a worthwhile means to improve your endurance.

Myth: Richer soil makes food richer in vitamins.

Truth: The nutritive value of a food is determined primarily by the heredity in its seed. Thus, if minerals that are demanded by the plant's heredity are missing from the soil, the plant simply will not grow. If such minerals are scant in the soil, fewer plants will grow. In other words, the farmer whose soil lacks what plants need will soon be out of business, for he will not have a crop.

Vitamins in our foods are manufactured in the plants themselves by genetically controlled processes. The very fact that a fruit or vegetable exists is evidence that it has those nutrients that are essential for its growth and that it has been able to synthesize the vitamins necessary for its metabolism.

There are trace minerals that accumulate in the plant as it grows (such as iodine). These may or may not be part of its own food needs. Soils high or low in iodine (or selenium) tend to produce plants that are high or low in these minerals. On the other hand, special techniques of cultivation, such as "organic" farming, do not solve this problem. It can be solved only by adding the necessary mineral element to the soil or the food.

What does this mean for "organic" foods? Simply that they have no food value beyond the values of ordinary supermarket foods ... except they usually cost more!

Myth: Extra vitamins and minerals will make you feel less tired.

Truth: In general, vitamins and minerals are not medicines. The confusion here comes from the knowledge that serious vitamin or mineral deficiencies lead to symptoms, and that restoring the missing nutrients to the diet relieves the symptoms. Once adequate vitamins and minerals are included in the diets of normal people, extras rarely have beneficial effect. The vast majority of illnesses that afflict Americans cannot be prevented or cured by extra vitamins and minerals. And neither can fatigue, or that general overall tired feeling.

Myth: Vitamin C tablets are great for warding off those winter colds.

Truth: The value of vitamin C in preventing colds is still controversial. Most nutrition experts note, however, that the massive doses recommended (up to 5,000 mg. in pill form a day) can cause diarrhea, excessive urination, and kidney and bladder stones. And they question its value in preventing colds. Until more conclusive evidence is available, the athlete need not consume more than the normal daily vitamin C requirement ... which is easily obtainable from four servings of fruits and vegetables.

As research continues, there will be more answers as to how much is too much of a vitamin, what the entire scope of usefulness of each vitamin is, and which medical conditions may respond well to vitamin therapy. In the meantime, athletes should know that elaborate testimonials, miraculous claims, and vitamins supposedly derived from exotic sources result from mere guesswork, confusion, and often, outright fraud.

Myth: High-fiber diets can cure many of your aches and pains.

Truth: Mark Twain once put to an end the rumor of his own death by remarking that the story was "greatly exaggerated." There are many times when scientists wish it were that easy to put a stop to the exaggerated fads built on legitimate discoveries or in-progress studies. A good case in point is the current furor over fiber. Dietary fiber, bran in particular, is being promoted as good for almost everything that ails you, from constipation to heart disease. High-fiber cookbooks are on the increase. So are the high-fiber foods on supermarket shelves.

Yet to the scientists who are investigating the effect of dietary fiber, the situation is far from clear. In fact, there are only two areas of general agreement.

A diet high in fiber plays a role in the prevention of constipation and diverticular disease (abnormal sacs or protusions on the walls of the intestines). On the other hand, dietary fiber by itself, probably has no effect on cancer of the colon or coronary heart disease, or other diseases of a less serious nature.

Before you buy a high-fiber supplement (like bran), examine your present diet. Food fiber comes in hundreds of different varieties, not just bran. For example, whole-wheat bread contains ample amounts of fiber. So does broccoli, raw cabbage, apples, pineapples, carrots, and whole kernel corn.

How much fiber should the average athlete include in his or her diet? Authorities differ in their recommendations. We know that intake of crude fiber among the American people is about four grams a day, compared with as much as 30 grams in some nonindustrialized countries. The answer for most people probably lies somewhere in between.

The best advice on fiber is . . . don't overdo it. A daily diet that is ample in fruits and vegetables as well as breads and cereals, should give you all you need of useful fiber. Supplementary crude fiber is best obtained from certain breakfast cereals, like Kellogg's All-Bran, Bran Buds, and Nabisco 100% Bran.

Myth: Athletes with digestive problems should consume yogurt each day.

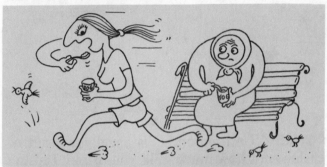

Truth: Yogurt is a fermented milk product and like all dairy products, it's an excellent source of protein and calcium. To say, however, that yogurt will help digestive problems is misleading. For those of you who have an allergic reaction to the lactose in milk (recent findings show that up to 75 percent of black athletes have this problem), then yogurt, since the fermentation process alters the lactose, may be helpful. The same thing can be said of buttermilk, which has almost equal nutritional value to that of yogurt and is considerably less expensive. In the 1950s and 1960s many health food faddists claimed that yogurt contained beneficial bacteria that assisted intestinal function. This has been proven false.

47

Myth: Stay away from milk because it causes "cottonmouth."

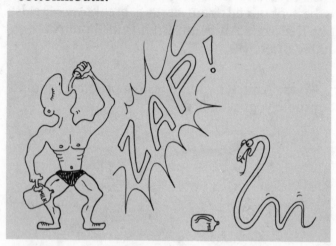

Truth: "Cottonmouth" is usually a result of tension, not how much milk you drink! Tension causes the salivary glands to decrease the flow of saliva. As a result, the mouth becomes dry and feels fuzzy. Water, ice, soft drinks, and chewing gum are effective in combating this condition.

Myth: Chemical additives to food are bad for you.

Truth: All of nutrition and all of life is chemistry. For example, an orange is a mixture of some 225 chemical compounds.

When you eat an orange, the orange is broken down to chemicals. What happens now is a process of picking and choosing. The chemicals that the body can use, it uses. Those it can't use, it eliminates.

The body doesn't choose between chemicals based upon whether they have chemical-sounding or natural-sounding names. Those prejudices exist in the mind, not the digestive system. The digestive system **does** care about two things: what the chemical is, and how much of it is there.

Recently, the term "chemical" has stood for what is man-made. And there has been the sad misunderstanding that what is "natural" is safe and good, and that what is man-made is potentially harmful. This has led to much needless worry and often to much exploitation of the consumer.

This does not mean that the U.S. Food and Drug Administration knows with absolute certainty that all chemical additives are safe. The important fact is that they do not know of any which are being used that are unsafe. Any knowledge of danger in an additive would result in its banishment from our food supply.

In reality, food additives are far safer than many natural components in foods. For example, carrots contain myristicin, a hallucinogen; radishes contain two substances which are goitiogens, they promote goiter by interfering with our use of iodine; potatoes contain solanine, which in great enough quantities can make you feel drowsy or paralyzed or cause breathing problems; shrimps contain some 40 to 170 or more parts per million of arsenic, and we all know what happens when we get too much of this chemical.

Similar chemicals can be found in all foods. Thus, if you consume too much of any **one** food, there's potential danger involved.

The whole point I'm trying to make is ... the foods found in the average home are not dangerous when consumed as a normal part of a balanced and varied diet. Eaten in moderation, they are all nutritious and safe.

Myth: Carbohydrates should be avoided by athletes.

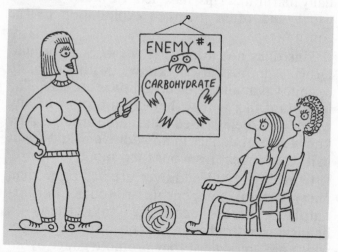

Truth: Since carbohydrates are really a basic fuel of the human body, nutritionists can scarcely believe that carbohydrates have recently gained the popular reputation of being harmful. When an athlete's intake of carbohydrates falls below about 50 to 100 grams a day, there is some real medical hazard ... especially since a typical athlete should consume over 350 grams a day.

Many of the most important body functions are designed to use carbohydrates as their only, or at least primary, fuel. For efficient operation, your brain must be powered by carbohydrates. The brain uses for its primary source of energy the sugar glucose, which comes mainly from the starch in the diet.

What if you don't eat enough carbohydrate for these body processes? Then the body actually takes proteins and certain parts of fats and converts them into carbohydrates. In other words, even if you go on a low-carbohydrate diet, your body's cells still get a lot of this nutrient. But you paid a high price in dollars and cents. You've been eating costly protein foods to get your indispensable carbohydrate, which you could have gotten from much less expensive items.

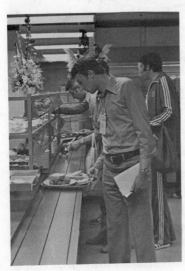

Carbohydrates (primarily in the form of breads, cereals, fruits, and vegetables) should be your primary source of energy.

Myth: Taking steroid drugs can be an effective way to gain muscular size and strength.

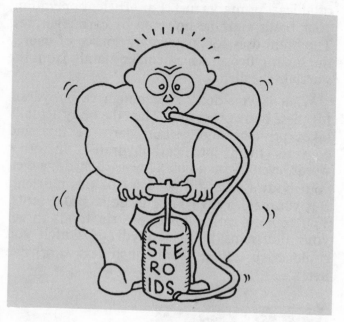

Truth: The most popular drugs used at the present time by athletes are the androgenic-anabolic steroids. **Androgenic** refers to the production of masculine characteristics, while **anabolic** relates to the conversion of food within a cell. These drugs are synthetic forms of testosterone and other male hormones. A few of the most common brand names are Dianabol, Winstrol, Anavar, Nilevar, Durabolin, and Methyltestosterone. In males it is **presumed** that the presence of androgens in increased quantities contributes to greater strength and muscle mass. As a result, athletes of all shapes and sizes (especially the marginal ones) have been consuming the drugs ... both legally (physician prescribed) and illegally (black market).

From a chemical standpoint, these drugs can not stimulate muscular growth. They cannot increase muscular strength. But, they can cause you to retain fluids (this accounts for the gain in bodyweight). And they can cause you to **think** you are stronger. This is basically a result of "placebo power," a well-known and documented phenomenon in medicine.

Don't minimize the power of placebos. Many studies consistently show that a placebo will produce the desired effect in about 30 percent of the patients when compared to real medicine. Other studies have demonstrated that placebos tend to be more effective when given in higher dosages, when given by injection rather than mouth, when it has an unpleasant taste, or when certain colors or shapes of pills are used.

Although the steroid drugs are **real** medicine, not just an indifferent substance, what they were clinically designed to do and what they are supposed to do (from the athlete's point of view) are worlds apart. The clinical purpose of androgenic-anabolic steroids is the treatment of some anemias, osteoporosis of the bone, chronic debilitating illness, and male hormone deficiencies. Once again, steroids do not make a healthy athlete bigger, stronger, or faster ... physiologically it's not possible!

The fact that the steroid drugs don't work from a chemical point of view would be relatively insignificant ... if there were no harmful side effects. Recently, a physician at a large New York hospital examined over 300 athletes who had been consuming large amounts of steroid drugs. He emphatically stated that he could detect clinical damage in 100 percent of the athletes up to six months after the drugs were discontinued, and permanent damage in more than 25 percent of the athletes. This damage was primarily in the form of one or more of the following: testicular atrophy, pituitary inhibition, prostate hypertrophy, fluid retention (high blood pressure), kidney damage (hardening of the kidney arteries), or impaired liver function (fibrosis).

All athletes using drugs in hopes that they will increase their performances would be wise to remember the following statement from Arthur Jones:

"There is no known drug that will improve the performance of a healthy athlete ... and there never will be such a drug; normal health being just that, normal ... super health, by definition, being impossible."

Myth: Athletes, because they are unique, do **not** require a balanced diet.

Truth: Athletes and non-athletes require a balanced diet composed of a wide variety of foods. Nutrition scientists have translated knowledge of the nutrient needs of people and the nutritive values of food into an easy-to-use guide for food selection.

This daily food guide sorts foods into four groups on the basis of their similarity in nutrient content. Each of the broad groups has a special contribution to make toward an adequate diet.

Daily Food Guide

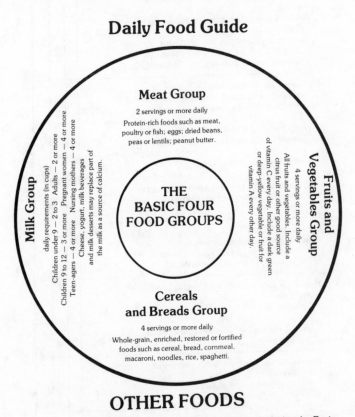

Meat Group

2 servings or more daily
Protein-rich foods such as meat, poultry or fish; eggs; dried beans, peas or lentils; peanut butter.

Milk Group

daily requirements (in cups)
Children under 9 — 2 to 3 Adults — 2 or more
Children 9 to 12 — 3 or more Pregnant women — 4 or more
Teen-agers — 4 or more Nursing mothers — 4 or more
Cheese, yogurt, milk beverages and milk desserts may replace part of the milk as a source of calcium.

THE BASIC FOUR FOOD GROUPS

Fruits and Vegetables Group

4 servings or more daily
All fruits and vegetables. Include a citrus fruit or other good source of vitamin C every day. Include a dark green or deep-yellow vegetable or fruit for vitamin A every other day.

Cereals and Breads Group

4 servings or more daily
Whole-grain, enriched, restored or fortified foods such as cereal, bread, cornmeal, macaroni, noodles, rice, spaghetti.

OTHER FOODS

To add variety and additional calories, other foods not specified in the Basic Four Food Groups may be used. Such foods include butter, margarine, oil, salad dressing, gravies, sauces, sugars, jams, jellies, candies, syrups, sweet desserts, sweetened and alcoholic beverages.

Food Selection Scorecard

Score your diet for each day using the points allowed for each food group. If your score is between 90 and 100, your food selection standard has been good; a score of 75 to 85 indicates a fair standard; a score below 75 is a low standard.

Points allowed (See basic-four food groups for serving size and substitutions.)	Maximum points for each group	Columns for daily check		
Milk (include cheese, ice cream, and milk used in cooking) Adults: 1 glass, 10 points; 1½ glasses, 15; 2 glasses, 20. Teen-agers and children 9 to 12: 1 glass, 5 points: 2 glasses, 10; 3 glasses, 15; 4 glasses, 20. Children under 9: 2 glasses, 15; 3 glasses, 20.	20			
Vegetables and fruits (serving = ½ cup) Vegetables: 1 serving, 5; 2 servings, 10. Potatoes may be included as one of these servings.	10			
Using 1 serving of dark green or deep yellow vegetable will earn you 5 extra points.	5			
Fruits: 1 serving, 5; 2 servings, 10.	10			
Using citrus fruit, raw cabbage, canned or raw tomatoes, berries, or melons gives 5 extra points.	5			
Cereals and breads Whole grain, enriched, or restored: Bread, rice, breakfast cereals, macaroni, etc.: 2 servings, 10 points; 4 servings, 15.	15			
Meat, eggs, fish, poultry, dried peas or beans, peanut butter: 1 serving, 10; 2 servings, 15.	15			
Using 1 serving liver or other organs gives 5 extra points.	5			
Total liquids (include milk, broth, tea, coffee, other beverages) Adults: 6 glasses, 3; 8 glasses, 5. Children: 4 glasses, 3; 6 glasses, 5.	5			
Eating a breakfast which included food from the meat or milk group. Do not count cream or bacon (except Canadian bacon) in this score.	10			
Daily score	100			

Part 2

Nutrients . . . What They Do and Where They Are Found

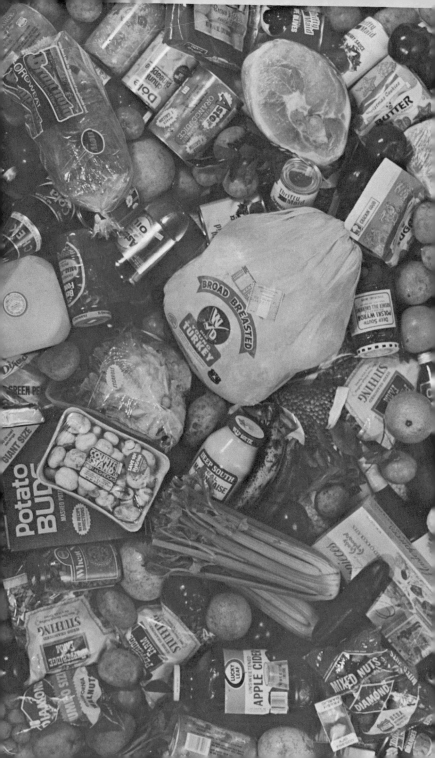

Nutrients ... What They Do and Where They Are Found

This section offers a convenient reference for those of you who want to know more about nutrition. It tells how proteins, carbohydrates, fats, minerals, vitamins, and water function in the body.

These facts will help you understand why athletes need a well-chosen variety of foods to be adequately nourished and healthy.

Proteins

All life requires protein. It is the chief tissue builder; the basic substance of every cell in the body.

Protein is made up of smaller units called amino acids. After foods are eaten, the proteins are broken down -- digested -- into amino acids which are then rearranged to form the many special and distinct proteins in the body.

The proteins in food are usually made up of 18 or more amino acids. The body can make its own supply of more than half of these. But the others must come ready-made from food and are called essential amino acids.

The amino acid makeup of a food protein determines its nutritive value. Proteins that supply all the essential amino acids in about the same proportions needed by the body are highest in value. Foods that provide good amounts of these top-ranking proteins best meet the body's needs. Generally these are foods of animal origin -- meat, fish, poultry, eggs, and milk.

Proteins from cereal grains, vegetables, and fruits do not provide as good an assortment of amino acids as animal proteins do, but they do supply valuable amounts of many amino acids. Proteins from legumes, especially the soybeans, and chickpeas, are almost as good as proteins from animal sources.

To have your daily meals rank well in protein quality, only a portion of the protein needs to come from animal sources. Combining cereal and vegetable foods with a little meat or other source of animal protein will improve the protein value of the meal. Examples of nourishing combinations are cereal with milk, rice with fish, spaghetti with meat sauce, vegetable stew with meat. Or you could simply have milk as a beverage along with foods of plant origin. It is a good idea to have some food from animal sources at each meal.

You need protein all through life for the maintenance and repair of body tissues. Children urgently need protein for normal growth.

Building of cells is only one of the roles of protein in the body. Among other functions, protein helps to:

- Make hemoglobin, the blood protein that carries oxygen to the cells and carries carbon dioxide away from the cells.
- Form antibodies that fight infection.
- Supply energy if carbohydrates and fats are not available.

Important amounts of protein are found in meat, poultry, fish, milk, cheese, eggs, dry beans, dry peas, and nuts.

Bread, cereals, vegetables, and fruits contain relatively smaller amounts of protein. However, the quantity of bread -- and perhaps of cereal -- eaten daily may be large enough to make these foods important sources.

Carbohydrates

Foods supply carbohydrates chiefly in three forms -- starches, sugars, and celluloses (fibrous materials). Starches and sugars are major sources of energy for humans. Celluloses furnish bulk in the diet.

Glucose, commonly called blood sugar, is the form in which starches and sugars are mainly used by cells to furnish energy for body processes and to support activity and growth.

Carbohydrates spare proteins by supplying energy, thereby saving protein for tissue building and repair and for other special jobs. Carbohydrates also help the body use fats efficiently.

Good sources of starch are grains (such as wheat, oats, corn, and rice), products made from grains (such as flour, macaroni, spaghetti, noodles, grits, breads, and breakfast cereals), potatoes, sweetpotatoes, and dry beans and peas.

Most other vegetables, fruits, and fruit juices contain smaller amounts of carbohydrate. In vegetables this is mainly in the form of starches; in fruits, it is chiefly sugars.

Cane and beet sugars, jellies, jams, candy and other sweets, honey, molasses, and syrups are concentrated sources of sugar.

Fruits, vegetables, and whole-grain cereals provide bulk for normal health of the intestinal tract.

Fats

Fats are concentrated sources of energy. Weight for weight, they give more than twice as much energy, or calories, as either carbohydrates or protein.

Everyone needs some fat. Primarily the fats supply energy, but they also carry the fat-soluble vitamins A, D, E, and K.

Fats also:
- Make up part of the structure of cells.
- Form a protective cushion around vital organs.

- Spare protein for body building and repair by providing energy.
- Supply an essential fatty acid, linoleic acid.

The body does not manufacture linoleic acid so it must be provided by food. It's found in valuable amounts in many oils that come from plants -- particularly corn, cottonseed, safflower, sesame, soybean, and wheat germ. These are referred to as "polyunsaturated" fats or oils. Margarines, salad dressings, mayonnaise, and cooking oils are usually made from one or more of these oils. Nuts contain less linoleic acid than most vegetable oils; among the nuts, walnuts rate quite high. Poultry and fish oils have more linoleic acid than other animal fats, which rank fairly low as sources.

In choosing your daily meals, it is best to keep the total amount of fat at a moderate level and to include some foods that contain polyunsaturated fats.

In cooking, fats add flavor and variety to many foods. Fats also make foods -- and meals -- satisfying because fats digest slowly and delay a feeling of hunger.

Common sources of fats are: butter, margarine, shortening, cooking and salad oils, cream, most cheeses, mayonnaise, salad dressing, nuts, and bacon and other fatty meats. Meats, whole milk, eggs, and chocolate contain some fat naturally. Many popular snacks, baked goods, and pastries and other desserts are made with fat or cooked in it.

Cholesterol

Cholesterol is a fat-like substance made in the body and found in every cell. It is a normal constituent of blood and tissues. In addition to the cholesterol made in the body, smaller amounts come from food. Cholesterol content of the diet is but one of many factors that influence the cholesterol level in blood.

Cholesterol is found only in foods of animal origin. It is not present in fruits, vegetables, cereal grains, legumes, or nuts, or in vegetable oils or other foods that come from plants. The highest concentrations of cholesterol are found in organ meats -- brain, liver, kidney, heart, sweetbreads, gizzards -- and in egg yolk. Shrimp is moderately high in cholesterol. Other foods of animal origin contain smaller quantities.

Mineral Elements

Many minerals are required by the body. They give strength and rigidity to certain body tissues, and help you with numerous vital functions.

Calcium

Calcium is the most abundant mineral element in the body. Teamed up with phosphorus, it is largely responsible for the hardness of bones and teeth. About 99 percent of the calcium in the body is found in these two tissues.

The small amount of calcium in other body tissues and fluids aids in the proper functioning of the heart, muscles, and nerves, and helps the blood coagulate during bleeding.

Milk is outstanding as a source of calcium. Appreciable amounts are contributed by cheese (especially the Cheddar types), ice cream, certain dark-green leafy vegetables (collards, kale, mustard greens, turnip greens), and canned salmon (if the bones are eaten).

Iodine

People who live away from the seacoast in areas where the soil is low in iodine sometimes fail to get an adequate supply of this mineral. Getting too little iodine can cause goiter, a swelling of the thyroid gland.

Iodized salt and seafoods are reliable sources of iodine. Regular use of iodized salt is the most practical way to assure enough iodine in your diet.

Iron

Iron is needed by the body in relatively small, but vital amounts. It combines with protein to make hemoglobin, the red substance of blood that carries oxygen from the lungs to body cells and removes carbon dioxide from the cells. Iron also helps the cells obtain energy from food.

Only a few foods contain much iron. Liver is a particularly good source. Lean meats, heart, kidney, shellfish, dry beans, dry peas, dark-green vegetables, dried fruit, egg yolk, and molasses also count as good sources. Whole-grain and enriched bread and cereals contain smaller amounts of iron, but when eaten frequently become important sources.

Frequent use of foods providing important amounts of iron is particularly encouraged for young children, preteen and teenage girls, and for women of childbearing age. Research shows these are the groups whose diets are most likely to be short in iron.

Other Essential Minerals

Two other minerals with vitally important functions are phosphorus and magnesium. Like calcium, they are found in largest amounts in bones and teeth. Among their other functions, they play an indispensable role in the body's use of food for energy.

Magnesium is found in good amounts in nuts, whole-grain products, dry beans, dry peas, and dark-green vegetables. Phosphorus is found in a variety of foods. If your meals contain foods that provide enough protein and calcium, you very likely will get enough phosphorus as well.

The other 10 or so essential minerals not discussed here that help keep the body functioning in a smooth and orderly fashion will usually be provided in satisfactory amounts by a well-chosen variety of foods as outlined in the Daily Food Guide.

Fluoride -- which helps protect teeth from decay -- may be an exception. During the years when teeth are being formed, drinking water that contains a proper amount of fluoride (either natural or added) will make teeth more resistant to decay.

Vitamins

Vitamins play a dynamic role in body processes -- they take part in the release of energy from foods, promote normal growth of different kinds of tissue, and are essential to the proper functioning of nerves and muscle.

A dozen or more major vitamins that food must provide have been identified. Ordinarily, you can get all the vitamins you need from a well-chosen assortment of everyday foods, such as is suggested in the Daily Food Guide.

Here is a summary of the vitamins -- including some of their functions and a list of foods that are dependable sources.

Vitamin A

Vitamin A occurs only in foods of animal origin. However, many vegetables and fruits, particularly the green and yellow ones, contain a substance called carotene that the body can change into vitamin A.

Liver is outstanding for vitamin A. Important amounts are also found in eggs, butter, margarine, whole milk, and cheese made with whole milk. Carotene is found in largest amounts in dark-green and deep-yellow vegetables and in deep-yellow fruits.

Vitamin D

Vitamin D is important in building strong bones and teeth because it enables the body to use the calcium and phosphorus supplied by food.

Few foods contain much vitamin D naturally. Milk with vitamin D added is a practical source. Small amounts of vitamin D are present in egg yolk, butter, liver; larger amounts occur in sardines, salmon, herring, and tuna.

Another source is the vitamin D produced by action of direct sunlight on the skin.

To supplement amounts from sunlight and food, vitamin D preparations may be prescribed by a physician for infants and young children.

Ascorbic Acid (Vitamin C)

Ascorbic acid helps form and maintain cementing material that holds body cells together and strengthens the walls of blood vessels. It also assists in normal tooth and bone formation and aids in healing wounds.

Citrus fruits -- oranges, grapefruit, lemons, and their juices -- and fresh strawberries are rich in ascorbic acid. Other important sources include tomatoes and tomato juice; broccoli; brussels sprouts; cabbage; cantaloupe; cauliflower; green peppers; some dark-green leafy vegetables such as collards, kale, mustard greens, spinach, turnip greens; potatoes and sweetpotatoes, especially when cooked in the jacket; watermelon.

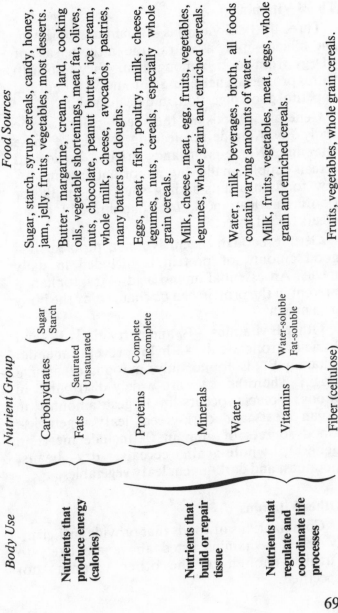

Body Use	Nutrient Group	Food Sources
Nutrients that produce energy (calories)	Carbohydrates — Sugar, Starch	Sugar, starch, syrup, cereals, candy, honey, jam, jelly, fruits, vegetables, most desserts.
	Fats — Saturated, Unsaturated	Butter, margarine, cream, lard, cooking oils, vegetable shortenings, meat fat, olives, nuts, chocolate, peanut butter, ice cream, whole milk, cheese, avocados, pastries, many batters and doughs.
Nutrients that build or repair tissue	Proteins — Complete, Incomplete	Eggs, meat, fish, poultry, milk, cheese, legumes, nuts, cereals, especially whole grain cereals.
	Minerals	Milk, cheese, meat, egg, fruits, vegetables, legumes, whole grain and enriched cereals.
	Water	Water, milk, beverages, broth, all foods contain varying amounts of water.
Nutrients that regulate and coordinate life processes	Vitamins — Water-soluble, Fat-soluble	Milk, fruits, vegetables, meat, eggs, whole grain and enriched cereals.
	Fiber (cellulose)	Fruits, vegetables, whole grain cereals.

The B Vitamins

Three of the B vitamins -- thiamin, riboflavin, and niacin -- play a central role in the release of energy from food. Among them, they also help with proper functioning of nerves, normal appetite, good digestion, and healthy skin.

Generally, foods in the meat group of the Daily Food Guide are leading sources of these vitamins. Whole-grain and enriched bread and cereals supply smaller but important amounts. A few foods are outstanding sources -- milk for riboflavin, lean pork for thiamin, and organ meats for all three.

Getting enough niacin is not a problem if a good amount of protein is included in daily meals. An essential amino acid -- tryptophan -- present in the protein can be changed by the body into niacin.

Other B vitamins -- B_6 and particularly B_{12} and folacin (folic acid) -- help prevent anemia. Vitamin B_{12} is found only in foods of animal origin. The other two are widely distributed in foods. Folacin occurs in largest amounts in organ meats and dark-green, leafy vegetables. Good sources of vitamin B_6 include meats in general, whole-grain cereals, dry beans, potatoes, and dark-green, leafy vegetables.

Other Vitamins

Combinations of foods that provide sufficiently for the vitamins listed above are likely to furnish enough of the other vitamins not specified.

Water

Water is essential for life. It ranks next to air, or oxygen, in importance. The body's need for water even exceeds its need for food. You can live for days, even weeks, without food, but only a few days without water.

About one-half to two-thirds of the body is made up of water. Water is the medium of body fluids, secretions, and excretions. It carries food materials from one part of the body to the other.

Also, water is the solvent for all products of digestion. It holds them in solution and permits them to pass through the intestinal wall into the bloodstream for use throughout the body. Water carries wastes from the body as well.

Some other roles of water are to:

- Regulate body temperature by evaporation through the skin and lungs.
- Aid digestion.
- Sustain the health of all cells.

It takes a regular and generous intake of water to perform all these jobs. The body gets water from many sources. The most obvious is the water you drink, but this often represents only a small part of total intake. Water also comes in beverages (coffee, tea, juice, soft drinks, milk) and soups. Foods, such as vegetables, fruits, meat, and even bread and dry cereals, contain some water. And water is formed when the body uses food for energy.

Estimating Caloric Requirements

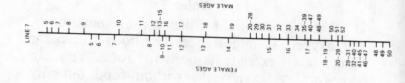

MALE AGES

FEMALE AGES

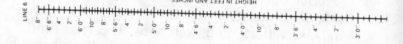

HEIGHT IN FEET AND INCHES

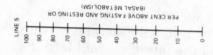

PER CENT ABOVE FASTING AND RESTING OR (BASAL METABOLISM)

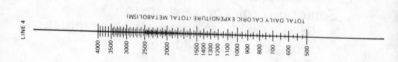

TOTAL DAILY CALORIC EXPENDITURE (TOTAL METABOLISM)

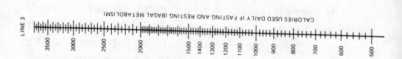

CALORIES USED DAILY IF FASTING AND RESTING (BASAL METABOLISM)

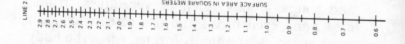

SURFACE AREA IN SQUARE METERS

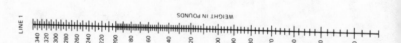

WEIGHT IN POUNDS

To determine the number of calories you burn in 24 hours, proceed as follows:

1. Using a pin as a marker, locate your actual weight on line 1.

2. Placing the edge of a ruler against the pin, move the other end to your height on line 6.

3. Remove the pin and place it at the point where the ruler crosses line 2.

4. Keeping the edge of the ruler firmly against the pin on line 2, move the right-hand edge to your age and sex on line 7.

5. Remove the pin and place it where the ruler crosses line 3. This gives you the calories used daily if you are resting and fasting.

6. To the basal calories thus determined, add the percentage above fasting and resting for your type of activity or lifestyle. For example, add 50 to 60 percent for manual laborers, active students, and athletes; 30 to 40 percent for typical Americans who participate in nothing more than light work; or 10 to 20 percent for people confined mostly to sitting activities. Leaving the pin in line 3, move the edge of the ruler to the right to the proper percentage on line 5. Where the ruler crosses line 4, you'll find the number of calories necessary to **maintain** your present weight.

Approximate Calories in Common Foods

	Portion	Calories
Meats		
Bacon, drained	2 slices	95
Beef, chuck	3 oz.	265
Beef, ground	3 oz.	245
Beef and vegetable stew	1 cup	250
Chicken, fried	1, 5 oz. leg	160
Frankfurter	1	125
Ham, baked	3 oz.	340
Pork chop	3 oz.	285
Fish		
Flounder	4 oz.	80
Salmon, canned	3 oz.	120
Tuna, canned	3 oz.	170
Dairy Products and Eggs		
Butter (or margarine)	1 tbsp.	100
Cheese, American	1 oz.	115
Cheese, cottage	1 oz.	25
Cream, whipped	1 tbsp.	50
Egg, boiled	1 large	75
Egg, scrambled	1 large	105
Milk, skim	1 cup	85
Milk, whole	1 cup	165
Fruits		
Apple, raw	1 medium	75
Apricots, dried	5 halves	50
Banana	1 medium	90
Grapefruit	½ medium	75
Orange	1 large	105
Orange juice, fresh	1 cup	110
Peach	1 medium	45
Pear	1 large	95
Vegetables		
Beans, baked	1 cup	325
Beans, string	1 cup	25
Beets	1 cup	70
Cabbage, raw	1 cup	25
Carrots, raw	1 medium	20

	Portion	Calories
Lettuce	2 leaves	5
Peas	1 cup	110
Potato, baked	1 medium	95
Potato chips	10 medium	110
Potato, french fried	8 pieces	155
Potato, mashed	1 cup	160
Tomato, raw	1 medium	30
Breads and Cereals		
Bread, white	1 slice	65
Bread, whole-wheat	1 slice	55
Corn flakes	1 cup	95
Macaroni, cooked	1 cup	210
Pancakes	1 medium	60
Rice, cooked	1 cup	205
Rolls, plain	1 medium	85
Rolls, sweet	1 medium	180
Spaghetti, cooked	1 cup	220
Salad Dressings		
French dressing	1 tbsp.	60
Mayonnaise	1 tbsp.	90
Thousand island	1 tbsp.	75
Candies and Desserts		
Cake, plain layer (icing)	2" wedge	320
Cake, pound	1 slice	130
Chocolate fudge	1, 1¼" sq.	115
Cookies, plain	1, 3" diameter	110
Doughnut, plain	1	135
Honey	1 tbsp.	60
Ice cream, vanilla	1 serving	165
Jams, jellies	1 tbsp.	50
Milk chocolate	1 bar	145
Pie, apple or berry	1/7, 9" pie	330
Sugar, brown	1 tbsp.	50
Sugar, granulated	1 tbsp.	40
Syrup, table	1 tbsp.	55

Part 3

How to Gain Bodyweight

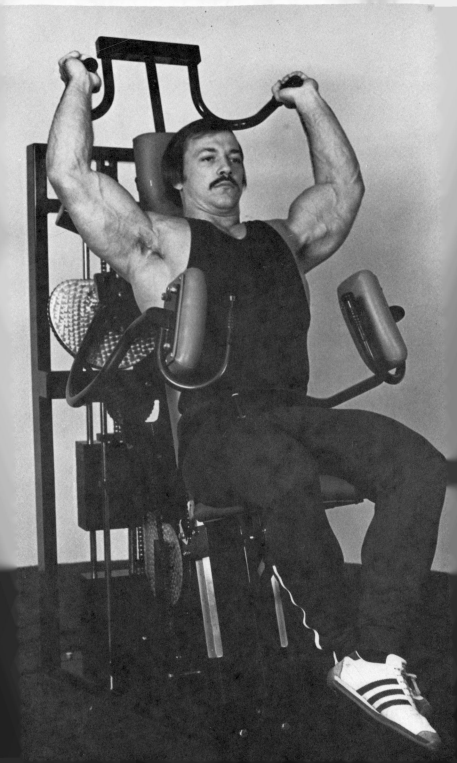

How to Gain Bodyweight

What's the most successful ad in the history of advertising ... an ad that has remained virtually unchanged for over 50 years? The answer is none other than Charles Atlas' sand-kicking ad!

Although Charles Atlas has been dead since 1972, his company has continued to prosper under the direction of his life-long friend and partner, Charles Roman.

"Of the 250,000 inquiries we get each year about our mail-order courses," said Mr. Roman in a recent telephone conversation, "the majority of the writers are interested in gaining weight -- solid weight -- in the right places!"

How widespread is the desire to gain weight? A recent Gallup Youth Survey found that among teenage boys (13-18 years old) 37 percent wanted to gain weight, 28 percent wanted to lose weight, and 35 percent were satisfied with their present weight. Among teenage girls, the picture is quite different. Two-thirds of the teenage girls questioned say they would like to lose weight (see table for complete details on next page).

Gallup Youth Survey
Do You Want to Gain or Lose Weight?

	Gain	Lose	Stay Same
NATIONWIDE	24%	47%	28%
Boys	37	28	35
13-15 years old	33	33	33
16-18 years old	40	24	36
Girls	12	66	21
13-15 years old	16	63	20
16-18 years old	8	70	22

Note: The survey results are based on a representative sample of 1,035 teenagers from across the nation, interviewed by telephone during the period June 22-July 8, 1977.

The above table shows that the desire to gain weight is primarily a male attitude, which seems to be more prevalent among boys in the older teen group.

The fact that teenage boys want to weigh more is not surprising to me. When I was 14 years of age, I sent away for Atlas' course ... as did many of you. But, I didn't stop with Atlas. In addition, I ordered barbells, dumbbells, springs, and weighted boots. Then, I spent ample amounts of money on various food supplements (high-protein powder, wheat germ oil, vitamin and mineral pills, desiccated liver tablets, etc.) since all the muscle-building magazines promoted them as being essential for results.

Was I rewarded for my efforts? Did I gain the solid bodyweight I desired?

Eventually I did gain some weight, most of which was in the form of fat (excess calories equals fat). And gradually over a five-year period of time, I did gain muscle, not from Atlas' "Dynamic Tension" exercise, but from a systematic program of progressive resistance exercise.

So, there continues to be an on-going interest among teenage boys in gaining weight. But for every boy that gets significant results, there're probably over a thousand that get little or no results to show for their efforts. Even for the very few who get some results, the results are usually not worth the price they have to pay!

Body Composition

The human body according to Dr. L. P. Novak, can be considered as a four-compartmental system:

Bodyweight = fat + extracellular water + muscle cells + bone minerals.

Of these four compartments, the ones most likely to show measurable increases or decreases are fat and muscle cells.

Generally speaking, body fat is composed of subcutaneous fat, depot fat, and essential fat. Subcutaneous fat consists of layers of fat found directly under the skin all over the body. It makes up the major percentage of fat in most individuals. Depot fat is usually deposited in the abdominal region in men and around the hips and thighs in women. Essential fat is necessary for the normal maintenance of the body. It makes up the covering of nerves, the membranes of cells, and cushions and protects many vital organs of the body.

There are also three types of muscle in the human body differing both in structure and function: skeletal, smooth, and cardiac. Skeletal muscles attach to bones and their contractions allow us to move. Smooth muscles are basically involuntary and make up our internal organs (stomach, intestines, gall bladder, etc.). Cardiac or heart muscle is unique in that it has spontaneous contractability and extremely rapid recovery.

On the one hand, the human body has a tremendous capacity to increase the size and number of subcutaneous and depot cells. Food calories over and above an individual's daily energy requirements lead to a slow but sure increase in body fat (3,500 calories equal a pound of fat).

On the other hand, the human body has a great (but lesser) capacity to increase the size of skeletal muscle cells. While calories are important in gaining muscle (600 calories in a pound of muscle), exercise is of far greater importance -- exercise that stimulates the muscles to grow larger and stronger.

Thus, when weight gain occurs in the human body (outside of the natural maturation process and pregnancy), what we are actually saying is that there is an increase in fat (subcutaneous and depot), muscle (skeletal), or both muscle and fat.

Muscle cells are active. Much of their time is spent contracting and stretching. Fat cells, however, are fairly inactive. They don't have nearly as many blood vessels to them as do muscle cells. Fat cells do not have much in the way of metabolic activity and can function on considerably less oxygen than our active muscle cells.

Fat does not contribute to muscular contraction. In fact, fat between muscle fibers acts as a friction brake and can actually impede the normal, relatively frictionless movement of lean muscle fibers during exercise. In the performance of most sports, muscles literally contribute everything, while fat contributes nothing!

As a result, most athletes would perform much better with a greater percentage of muscle mass and a smaller percentage of body fat. Outside of long-distance swimming and Sumo wrestling, I can't think of any sport where additional body fat would be an advantage.

The human body contains 434 skeletal muscles. These muscles are our only means of movement. Without muscles, we would be little more than vegetables. From a logical point of view, any time an athlete increases his muscle mass to bodyweight ratio, he improves his movement potential.

How the Body Gains Muscle Mass

Muscle growth consists of three parts. **One,** there must be growth stimulation within the body itself at the basic cellular level. After puberty, this is best accomplished by high-intensity exercise. **Two,** the proper nutrients must be available for the stimulated cells. But providing large amounts of nutrients, in excess of what the body requires, will not do anything to promote growth of muscle fibers. The growth machinery within the cell must be turned on. Muscle stimulation must always precede nutrition. If an athlete has stimulated muscular growth by high-intensity exercise, then his muscles will grow on almost any reasonable diet, given that his body is given sufficient time. **Three,** sufficient time, time spent resting and recovering, is the final requirement for muscular growth.

Why, then, do so many athletes who are trying to build muscle mass, consume large amounts of protein foods? Because at some point in time they have heard that ... "muscles are made up of protein" ... and ... "to build muscles, you need to eat lots of protein." This is simply not true! Only 22 percent of a muscle is protein. Most of muscle is water (70 percent).

In other words, there are about 100 grams of protein, a small amount of fat, a lot of water, and around 600 calories in a pound of muscle. Thus, if an athlete stimulated a pound of muscle growth over a week's period of time, he would need to consume an extra 14 grams of protein and 86 calories each day. This is not much in the way of additional food, if any, since the typical athlete probably consumes three times as much protein as he needs a day.

The chemical reactions inside a growing muscle are much more complicated than just exercising, eating, and resting. High-intensity muscular contraction results in the formation of a chemical called creatine. The creatine stimulates the muscle to form more myosin, one of the contraction proteins within the muscle fiber. Thus, contraction of the muscle fiber produces creatine, which in turn causes the muscle to form more myosin, which enables it to undergo stronger contractions. This in turn causes the production of more creatine, and around we go again.

Creatine has been identified as the messenger substance that turns on the RNA (ribonucleic acid) processing line to produce muscle growth. The RNA molecules within a specialized compartment of the cell literally act as an assembly line and hook together various combinations of amino acids, sometimes in combination with complex sugars and fats to form different compounds that result in the increased size of certain muscle cells. Remember, an athlete must stimulate growth through high-intensity exercise, then provide the proper nutrients, and rest.

Training Programs to Gain Muscle Mass and Lose Body Fat ... At the Same Time

Gaining muscle and losing fat at the same time are accomplished by brief, infrequent, high-intensity exercise to stimulate growth in the major muscle groups combined with a well-balanced, reduced-calorie diet. The lower-calorie diet (about 500 calories below maintenance level) causes a gradual decrease in body fat. The high-intensity exercise causes a gradual increase in muscle mass. For the record, research with animals has shown that muscular growth can occur in rats fed no calories, just water, if they were exercised properly beforehand. Evidently, since a pound of fat contains 3,500 calories and a pound of muscle contains only 600 calories, the body can convert fat into the necessary raw materials to produce muscle mass -- given, of course, that the muscles are first stimulated to grow through high-intensity exercise.

What is high-intensity exercise? The words "high intensity" applied to exercise simply mean selecting a movement that involves a heavy overload and then performing as many repetitions as possible of this movement. For muscle-building purposes, high-intensity exercise is usually performed with barbells or weight machines like Nautilus or Universal. See the photos and data on the following pages.

A well-rounded program would consist of four to six exercises for the lower body and six to eight exercises for the upper body. One set of 8 to 12 repetitions, with as much weight as possible, should be performed every other day, or three times a week. Always add more resistance (about five percent) when 12 or more repetitions can be executed in good form.

Good form requires that all repetitions be moved in a slow, smooth manner. No throwing or jerking movements should be used. And special attention should be given to lowering the resistance (eccentric contraction). A review of related literature shows that for building muscular size and strength, lowering the resistance is more important than raising the resistance. As an example, if it takes two seconds to raise a weight, then it should take four seconds, or twice as long, to lower the same weight. All in all, it should take an athlete about one minute to complete a set of 10 repetitions in good form.

The following exercises, grouped by muscle group and equipment, are applicable to most strength-training programs:

Muscle Group	Barbells/ Dumbbells	Universal Gym	Nautilus Machines
Buttocks/ Lower Back	Squat Stiff-Legged Deadlift	Leg Press Hyperextension	Hip and Back Squat Leg Press
Quadriceps	Squat	Leg Extension Leg Press	Leg Extension Squat Leg Press
Hamstrings	Squat	Leg Curl Leg Press	Leg Curl Squat Leg Press
Calves	Calf Raise	Toe Press on Leg Press	Calf Raise on Multi Exercise Toe Press on Leg Press
Latissimus dorsi	Bent-Over Rowing Bent-Armed Pullover Stiff-Armed Pullover	Chin-Up Pulldown on Lat Machine	Pullover Behind Neck Torso/Arm ChinUp on Multi Exercise
Trapezius	Shoulder Shrug Dumbbell Shoulder Shrug	Shoulder Shrug	Neck and Shoulder Rowing Torso
Deltoids	Press Press Behind Neck Upright Rowing Forward Raise Side Raise with Dumbbells	Seated Press Upright Rowing	Double Shoulder 1. Lateral Raise 2. Overhead Press Omni Shoulder Rowing Torso
Pectoralis Majors	Bench Press Dumbbell Fly	Bench Press Parallel Dip	Double Chest 1. Arm Cross 2. Decline Press
Biceps	Standing Curl	Curl Chin-Up	Compound Curl Biceps Curl Omni Biceps Chin-Up on Multi Exercise
Triceps	Triceps Extension with Dumbbells	Press Down on Lat Machine	Compound Triceps Triceps Extension Omni Triceps Parallel Dip on Multi-Exercise
Forearms	Wrist Curl	Wrist Curl	Wrist Curl on Multi Exercise
Abdominal/ Obliques	Sit-Up Side Bend with Dumbbells	Sit-Up Leg Raise	Sit-Up on Multi-Exercise Leg Raise on Multi-Exercise Side Bend on Multi-Exercise
Neck	Neck Bridge (dangerous)	Neck Harness	4-Way Neck Rotary Neck Neck and Shoulder

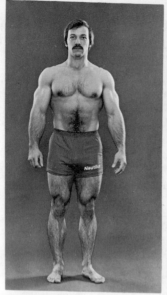 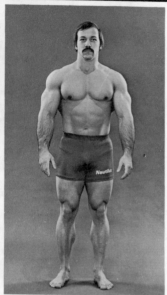

Oct. 15, 1977 → 10 weeks → Dec. 24, 1977
186 pounds   later   206 pounds

High-intensity exercise, not food consumption, is the key to gaining muscle mass. In order to prove this point, 26 year old Casey Viator participated in a controlled 10-week program of diet and high-intensity exercise.

Casey's food intake was limited to 1,800 calories a day (three, 600-calorie meals) for the entire 10-week period. Why only 1,800 calories a day? Because according to the table on page 72, at 186 pounds, Casey's basal metabolic requirements were calculated at approximately 1,800 calories. Incidentally, this was about half as many calories as he ordinarily consumed each day.

The exercise program that Casey adhered to consisted of 12 basic exercises performed on Nautilus machines. Each exercise was carried to the point of momentary muscular failure. Anytime 12 or more repetitions were performed in good style, the resistance was increased by approximately five percent at the next workout. Casey trained three days a week and each workout lasted less than 30 minutes.

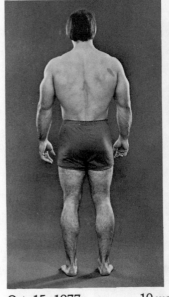 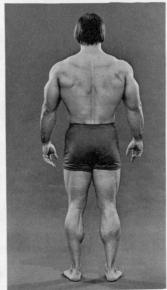

Oct. 15, 1977   10 weeks   Dec. 24, 1977
186 pounds   later   206 pounds

From the photos above, you can see Casey's progress. On the 12 basic exercises, Casey's strength increased an average of 28 percent per exercise. As a muscle gets stronger, its size and mass increases in almost direct proportion. Thus, his bodyweight went from 186 to 206, a gain of 20 pounds, or 2 pounds a week.

Putting on 20 pounds of muscle mass requires some calories, 12,000 to be exact, since there are 600 calories in a pound of muscle. So, in order for Casey Viator to build 20 pounds of muscle in 10 weeks, his body had to draw on his fat stores as a source of calories. Since there are approximately 3,500 calories in a pound of fat, Casey must have lost 3.43 pounds of body fat -- in addition to gaining 20 pounds of muscle mass. By closely observing the photos, you can see that Casey definitely has less fat in the second set of pictures.

The next two pages show some of the exercises that Casey performed.

Hip extension

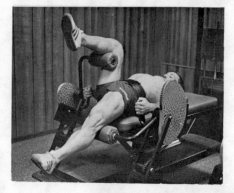

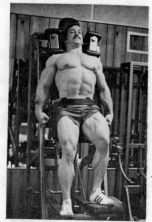

Squat

Leg extension

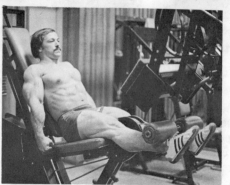

Calf raise

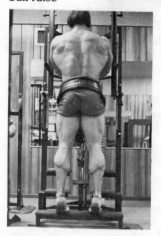

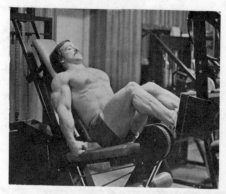

Leg press

Biceps curl

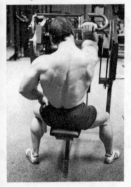

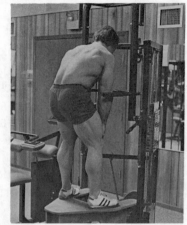

Deadlift

Overhead press

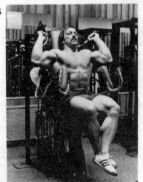

Pullover

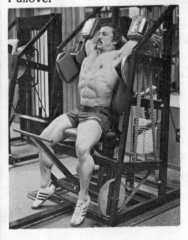

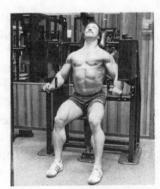

Neck extension

High-Calorie Diets

Many coaches think they have athletes who are under fat. In my opinion, these athletes are probably under muscled rather than under fat. I can't remember ever seeing an athlete that I considered to be under fat. Occasionally you do see teenage athletes that have high metabolic rates and high caloric requirements. If this is the case, the following guidelines can be used in developing high-calorie diets:

APPROXIMATE NUTRIENT CONTENT OF DAILY MEAL SCHEDULE

Approximate Calories	FAT		PROTEIN		CARBOHYDRATE	
	Grams	% Total Calories	Grams	% Total Calories	Grams	% Total Calories
2,500	70	28	79	13	374	59
3,750	105	28	118	13	561	59
5,000	140	28	158	13	748	59

TOTAL SERVINGS OF FOODS IN DAILY MEAL SCHEDULES

Approximate Calories	Whole Milk	Meat or Equivalent	Fruit	Veg.	Bread	Other
2,500	3 cups	5 ounces	6 ser.	2 ser.	8 ser. 4 with jelly	2 desserts 2 tsp. oil
3,750	4½ cups	7½ ounces	9 ser.	3 ser.	12 ser. 6 with jelly	3 desserts 3 tsp. oil
5,000	6 cups	10 ounces	12 ser.	4 ser.	16 ser. 8 with jelly	4 desserts 4 tsp. oil

Perhaps you are thinking that it might be difficult for an athlete to consume 5,000 calories a day and it would if he stuck to three meals a day. The listing below indicates how 5,000 calories can be consumed by eating three meals as well as three snacks each day. Of course, this sample diet is only offered as a guideline. You may want to substitute ice cream, fruit juice, popcorn, or cookies in the snack area. There are many foods that can be substituted for those listed.

Example Meal Schedule for 5,000 Calories

1. Breakfast
   - 2 cups milk
   - 3 ounces meat
   - 2 servings of fruit
   - 2 servings of bread
   - 2 servings of bread with jelly
2. Mid-morning snack
   - 2 servings of fruit
   - 2 servings of bread with jelly
3. Lunch
   - 2 cups milk
   - 3 ounces meat
   - 2 servings of fruit
   - 2 servings of vegetables
   - 3 servings of bread
   - 2 desserts
   - 2 teaspoon oil
4. Afternoon snack
   - 2 servings of fruit
   - 2 servings of bread with jelly
5. Dinner
   - 2 cups milk
   - 4 ounces meat
   - 2 servings of fruit
   - 2 servings of vegetables
   - 3 servings of bread
   - 2 desserts
   - 2 teaspoon oil
6. Evening snack
   - 2 servings of fruit
   - 2 servings of bread with jelly

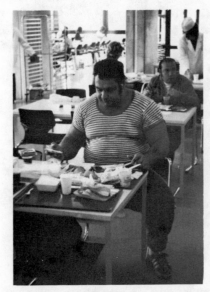

Many athletes who consume high-calorie diets for extended periods of time eventually end up with an obesity problem. This is certainly the case with the Russian athlete, 345-pound Vasily Alexeev. Remember, calories do count -- every one of them! Consume more than your body requires and your body will gradually get fatter.

In summary, the concept of gaining "weight" is misleading. What athletes and coaches should be concerned about is increasing skeletal muscle mass and decreasing body-fat stores. Both of these goals can be accomplished through high-intensity, progressive exercise along with a reasonable, mixed diet.

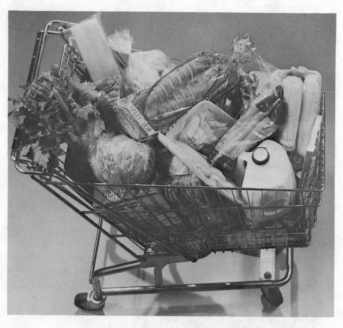

The basic factor in optimum nutrition for athletes is the daily selection of a wide variety of foods . . . which foods can still be conveniently purchased at your local supermarket.

Conclusion

The well-known generalization, "If a little is good, more is better," does **not** apply to nutrition. But the concept, "A little knowledge is a dangerous thing," certainly does apply.

Athletes need a wide variety of food because no single food contains all the necessary nutrients. In other words, there are no super or magic foods. And neither are there junk nor bad foods. Any food can be **good** if it is mixed in moderation with a variety of other foods, or any food can be **bad** if it is exclusively consumed.

In the long run, athletes would do well to realize that victory probably depends more on **individual potential** and **quality of coaching** than on nutritional factors.

Bibliography

"Bread: You Can't Judge a Loaf by Its Color." **Consumer Reports** 41:256-260, May 1976.

Darden, Ellington. "Positive and Negative Work" (part 2), **Scholastic Coach** 45:6-12, October 1975.

Darden, Ellington. **Nutrition and Athletic Performance.** Pasadena, California: The Athletic Press, 1976.

Darden, Ellington. **Strength-Training Principles.** Winter Park, Florida: Anna Publishing, 1977.

"Diet Crazes." **Newsweek** 90:66-77, December 19, 1977.

Gallup, George. "Do You Want to Gain or Lose Weight," **The Montgomery County Daily Courier (Conroe, Texas),** October 29, 1977.

Hall, Richard L. "Safe at the Plate," **Nutrition Today** 12:6-9, 28-31, November 1977.

"How Nutritious Are Fast-Food Meals?" **Consumer Reports** 40:278-281, May 1975.

How to Feed Your Family to Keep Them Fit and Happy . . . No Matter What. New York: Golden Press, 1972.

Howe, Phyllis Sullivan. **Basic Nutrition in Health and Disease.** Philadelphia: W. B. Saunders Co., 1976.

"Is Vitamin C Really Good for Colds?" **Consumer Reports** 41:68-70, February 1976.

Labuza, Theodore P. **The Nutritional Crisis: A Reader.** St. Paul: West Publishing Co., 1975.

Lamb, Lawrence E. **Metabolics.** New York: Harper and Row, 1974.

Mayer, Jean. "Liquid Protein: The Last Word on the 'Last Chance' Diet," **Family Health** 10:40-41, January 1978.

"McDonald's vs. Kentucky Fried: Rating the Fast-Food Chains." **Family Circle** 90:36, 40, 42, August 23, 1977.

National Research Council, Food and Nutrition Board: Recommended Dietary Allowances. Eighth revised edition. Washington, D. C., National Academy of Sciences, 1974.

Nelson, Ralph A. "What Should Athletes Eat? Unmixing Folly and Facts," **Physician and Sportsmedicine** 3:67-72, November 1975.

Novak, L. P. "Analysis of Body Compartments," in **Fitness, Health, and Work Capacity** (edited by L. A. Larson). New York: Macmillan, 1974.

Nutrition Labeling: How It Can Work for You. Bethesda, Maryland: The National Nutrition Consortium, Inc., 1975.

Scrimshaw, Nevin S., and Young, Vernon R. "The Requirements of Human Nutrition," **Scientific American** 235:50-64, September 1976.

Steben, R. E.; Wells, J. C.; and Harless, I. L. "Testing the Effects of Bee Pollen," **Track Technique** 64:2046-47, June 1976.

"Those Best-Seller Diets: Do They Really Work?" **Good Housekeeping** 185:292-300, November 1977.

Vitale, Frank. **Individualized Fitness Programs,** Englewod Cliffs, N. J.: Prentice-Hall, Inc., 1973.

"Vitamin E: What's Behind All Those Claims for It?" **Consumer Reports** 38:60-66, January 1973.

"Yogurt: Will it Keep You Fit?" **Consumer Reports** 43:7-12, January 1978.